DR. DAVE'S
THE LIT⁻

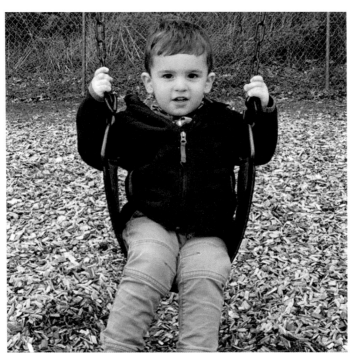

Figure 1 "Little Jeffrey"

To Tyla & Myles,
wishing you lots of good health,
happiness, & quiet nights!!

Dr. Dave

3-25-2020

Table of Contents

THE LITTLE JEFFREY BOOK

(What keeps parents and pediatricians awake at night)

INTRODUCTION

Deciding to retire was not an easy decision. Middle of the night phone calls were not as easy for me to address as they were when I was younger. When my "good ear" was down on the pillow at night, I would have to rely on my wife Nancy to wake me to answer the phone. Mid-day naps were looking more attractive and my hearing was getting more difficult in noisy environments. The introduction of electronic medical records led to two carpel tunnel surgeries. I found myself spending most of my time in the office dealing with the computer rather than with patients. As much as I hated to admit it, I knew the time had come.

What about the many years of acquired knowledge and 40 years of experience helping families with their newborns and children?

I felt bad knowing that I would be retiring just before the birth of my nephew Jeff and his wife Jessica's new baby. I took care of Jeff from birth to adulthood but now I wasn't there to help him with his own child. I became acutely aware of this as their questions arose with the inevitable concerns.

Their new son was also named Jeffery. Thanks to "little Jeffrey" I realized the time had come for me to put to print years of advice that I would give to parents for some of the more common and worrisome situations. So, this is dedicated to "Little Jeffrey".

Now I can catch up on my sleep and even take the occasional nap. Although I may not be responding to emergencies or answering calls in the middle of the night, I'm not quite ready to fully hang up my hat yet.

With pen in hand or rather fingers on the keyboard, I'd like to share some of the advice I used to give parents for some of their more common concerns, especially for those things that keep them and myself up at night.

The purpose of this writing is to share those night-time experiences and discussions made with concerned parents. It is not intended to be a medical reference. There are several excellent resources already in publication, particularly those of The American Academy of Pediatrics which can be found at the AAP.org website.

It is my hope that this may help to ease some of the worries and sleepless nights that go along with parenting.

Part I: Common Concerns and Illnesses

Ear Infections

" MY CHILD HAS ALREADY HAD 3 EAR INFECTIONS THIS WINTER. AM I DOING ANYTHING TO CAUSE THEM? LIKE GETTING WATER IN HIS EAR? IS THERE ANYTHING I SHOULD DO DIFFERENTLY?"

Ear infections (i.e. "middle" ear infections, otitis media) are typically associated with "colds" (i.e. "URI's" /upper respiratory infections). The cold viruses create an environment that makes it easier for bacteria to grow in. These bacteria work their way up from the nasal passages and back of the throat into the middle ear by way of the eustachian tube.

An intact eardrum (tympanic membrane) prevents water from entering the middle ear so that even very dirty water cannot enter the middle ear to cause an inner ear infection. On the other hand, it can contribute to "swimmer's ear" which is an infection of the ear canal referred to as otitis externa. Water gets trapped in the ear canal, often associated with pre-existing wax, it allows bacteria to grow, infecting the skin of the ear canal, causing an external infection.

The average child gets one cold per month during the fall and winter months. Considering most colds will last from 7-10 days, at times up to 2 weeks, half of the winter is spent fighting off common "colds".

With middle ear and sinus infections being very common secondary infections, it can seem as though the winter is one long continuous infection.

Since infants and young children have not yet built up immunity to common infections, this becomes a very common scenario amongst even healthy children.

Some children can inherit a middle ear anatomy which makes it easier for bacteria to make their way in and cause infection. Often their parents say, "I was the same way when I was his or her age".

On the other hand, there are those children that have problems with their immune system affecting their ability to fight infection (immunodeficiencies). Besides ear infections they tend to get infections that the average child does not get such as recurrent pneumonias.

The best way to prevent recurrent ear infections is to minimize potential exposure to other sick children. This is easier said than done. Some children are fortunate and hardly ever get sick no matter what their exposures are. This is not the case for most.

Well intended activities to promote development and socialization might be best deferred to those months when germs are much less prevalent like late spring and summer. For the great majority of families, day care is a necessity. Very few have the luxury of a stay at home parent, a dedicated grandparent or a live-in nanny. The upside to this is that by the time these children are ready to enter kindergarten or first grade, they are more immune to common infections and less likely to lose time from school due to illness.

Keeping up to date with immunizations at their recommended schedules is one of the best things a parent can do to help protect their children from becoming ill, especially during the most vulnerable ages of infancy and preschool years. Vaccines such as HIB, PVC13, and PREVNAR help build up immunity against some of the deadliest strains of bacteria that not only cause ear infections but are capable of life-threatening complications. Flu vaccine can also help since a significant percentage of children that get the flu develop secondary ear infections as well.

"HOW MANY EAR INFECTIONS ARE TOO MANY AND WHEN SHOULD A PARENT BE CONCERNED? WHEN SHOULD A CHILD GET TUBES AND SHOULD PARENTS BE CONCERNED ABOUT THE USE OF ANTIBIOTICS?"

Ear infections are extremely common in young children, especially toddlers and pre-school children.

Occasionally some ear infections resolve spontaneously, but most do not and without treatment they would require close office monitoring. Without close monitoring, worsening could go undetected leading to a ruptured eardrum (perforation of the tympanic membrane) or spreading beyond the middle ear into the blood (sepsis), lungs (pneumonia), or nervous system (meningitis). Complications can start to develop without obvious symptoms. The majority of ear infections are best treated with antibiotics. They should be rechecked following treatment or at any point in which a child's condition seems to be worsening.

Some infections prove to be resistant to an initial course of treatment and may require a different antibiotic or a more prolonged course of treatment with antibiotics. When ear infections completely resolve but then immediately return each and every time antibiotics are stopped, further evaluation is indicated to rule out a problem with the child's immune system.

It is not unusual to have residual sterile middle ear fluid (also known as a sterile effusion or serous otitis media) after ear infections have responded to an antibiotic. Although the fever, pain and inflammation of the eardrum are gone, sterile fluid often persists usually resolving spontaneously in 2 or 3 wks. Occasionally this fluid proves to be good food for more bacteria and leads to another infection.

Tubes: At times the fluid may persist for more than three months. Fluid lasting that long becomes very thick and viscous like cold molasses or glue creating what is called a *"glue ear"*. A glue ear is not likely to resolve spontaneously. It typically requires draining by means of *"tubes"* (referred to as *bilateral myringotomy and tubes*) inserted into the eardrum to restore hearing. As a secondary benefit, children typically have fewer or no further ear infections with tubes. *More than 3 ear infections in the winter*, especially during the fall or earlier months of the winter can also be an indication for tubes.

Although most children see a great improvement if the frequency of ear infections following tube insertions, it is still possible to get an ear infection (typically noted by a *draining ear*).

Having tubes inserted is a surgical day care procedure requiring very brief sedation/anesthesia. There are very rare but real risks to having this done.

The tubes usually stay in place 6-12 months then fall out spontaneously but occasionally much sooner. It may *not* be a good idea to undergo this procedure in late spring or summer when infections are much less common. The tubes could fall out prematurely and not be present when they are really needed in the fall and winter when infections reemerge. Summer also poses the potential problem of getting water in the ears which should be avoided when tubes are present. Persistent ear infections during the summer months are not very common, making fall and winter months the typical times of the year for this procedure.

On occasion the tubes do not spontaneously fall out as expected after a year or so and may necessitate removal by an ENT (Ears, Nose and Throat) physician. On rare occasion a persistent hole will remain in the ear drum (*tympanic membrane perforation*). This acts like a persistent tube. Although this has the same benefits of having a tube, it may lead to hearing loss and medical complications. Fortunately, most perforations will often close on their own given sufficient time.

***Treating ear infections* with antibiotics** is important in preventing serious complications. It is important to take prescription antibiotics for the full course, as directed, without skipping doses. Otherwise an incompletely treated infection could re-emerge several days later only to appear as a "new" infection.

Taking probiotics can help avoid significant secondary diarrhea. Treating initially with one of the "strongest" antibiotics is not always best as it can lead to resistant bacteria and increase risks of developing serious complications such as colitis from the bacteria *clostridium difficile (c. diff)*.

"What should I do if my child wakes up crying with ear pain?"

This is a common call to a pediatrician in the middle of the night. One can only imagine the desperate feeling a parent has when their child is crying or screaming with pain in the middle of the night. Making matters worse, this may be accompanied by a high fever. Every parent wishes there could be some antibiotic that could be administered in the middle of the night that would quickly make things better. Unfortunately, even if a child were given an antibiotic injection right then and there, it would not quickly make the pain go away.

The onset of pain occurs with stretching and bulging of the eardrum when an ear infection suddenly hits. Despite the initial severity of pain, it is not uncommon to see the same child in the morning, untreated, sitting up and smiling with no pain, only to be found to have a fiery red bulging eardrum.

Why is that? It would seem that most of the pain is generated with the initiation the actual stretching out of the eardrum. Subsequently the pain subsides. This could lead a parent to the false impression that they made it through the night ok and now there is no longer a need to see the doctor. Unfortunately, the infection can then progress and potentially into a complication. Days later a draining ear may develop when the eardrum ruptures.

So, what to do in the middle of the night? Treat the pain. If the situation can be temporized and be seen in your doctor's office the first thing in the morning, you might avoid what would otherwise seem like a very long night in the emergency room.

Relieving the pain:

1. Acetaminophen (Tylenol) every 4 hrs. up to 5 doses/24 hrs.

Caution: read label closely. Infant drops 80 mg/ml, children's liquid 160 mg/5ml, chewable 160 mg/tab. Correct dose is 10-15 mg/kg/dose. (Note: 2.2 lbs./kg).

2. *Ibuprofen* (Advil/Motrin) every 8 hrs. at 10 mg/kg/dose. *Read the product label closely*: infant drops 50mg/1.25 ml, children's liquid 100mg/5ml, chewable 100 mg/tab. Liquid and drops are absorbed and work the fastest.

These 2 medications can be staggered roughly 2 hrs. apart. Use caution when giving medications together at the same time. There is a risk of provoking vomiting making the situation appear much worse. An unnecessary trip to the Emergency Room might otherwise have been avoided.

Another measure that can be helpful is applying a moderately hot moist washcloth, folded into a compress over the ear. The moist heat helps to ease the stretching of the eardrum and helps soothe the pain. You can also try to relieve middle ear pressure by way of the *eustachian tube*. This is the tube that regulates middle ear pressure with atmospheric pressure. It connects the middle ear to an area behind the nasal passages above the soft palate.

Compare this to the pressure created when changing altitude in an

airplane or going down a mountain. It can be relieved by pinching your

nose, then trying to blow through it followed by swallowing. The effect

is feeling your ears "pop" as the pressure is relieved.

The same effect can potentially be obtained by trying to open the

nasal passages and the eustachian tube with the administration of

decongestant nose drops. These are available OTC (phenylephrine

0.125% in children 2-6 years old, 0.25% for 6-12 years old). Administer

1-3 drops and 2-4 drops respectively, every 2-4 hrs. intranasally, not to

exceed 3 days.

Lots of "TLC' can have a calming effect and also help buy a little

time while the eardrum is stretching out. If the child remains

inconsolable, or if the fever does not come down with simple measures,

then it's time to proceed to the emergency room.

Rashes

Rashes (non-specific and hive-like), are very common in young children. Often occurring coincidentally during a course of antibiotics. Most are non-specific viral *exanthems* and not a reaction to an antibiotic. These are rashes due to viruses not easily identified by a distinctive appearance such as measles or chickenpox. They are often the cause of the upper respiratory infection which led to an ear infection. Many viruses are capable of doing this.

With so many causes of rashes in children, it becomes commonplace for a rash to appear while taking antibiotics. It can be difficult to conclude that a rash is an allergic reaction to an antibiotic or not. Many antibiotic "allergies" are actually rashes due to other causes. They merit office evaluation and at times allergy testing rather than unnecessarily excluding use of an antibiotic when it could prove lifesaving in the future.

Before considering tubes, it is worth every effort to minimize potential exposures to other contagious individuals and children. Also consider possible problems with one's ability to fight infection, especially if there have been unusual infections such as recurrent pneumonias, fungal infections and uncommon skin infections.

If after addressing these issues frequent courses of antibiotics are still necessary, or severe secondary side effects from antibiotics, or multiple antibiotic allergies develop, seeing an otolaryngologist (ear, nose and throat-ENT specialist) for further evaluation and possible tubes (bilateral myringotomy and tubes) is indicated.

Another consideration is environmental *allergies* such as pollen, dust and pets. The congestion and mucus they produce provide ideal conditions for bacteria to grow. This can lead to secondary sinus and middle ear infections.

Identifying the specific cause of allergies (*allergens*) makes it easier to avoid or minimize exposure to them, hopefully lessening secondary infections.

Quite often children with environmental allergies are allergic to not one but numerous allergens. They tend to be very sensitive individuals overall and are referred to as *"atopic"*. They are prone to rashes particularly *eczema (atopic dermatitis)* and not infrequently also have asthma.

Dust control measures can be helpful. Avoiding dust collectors, utilizing a HEPA filter in the child's bedroom, and keeping pets out of the bed and bedroom, can be a big help. Frequent changing of central air/ forced hot air furnace filters is important. OTC antihistamines and nasal steroid sprays can provide good control measures.

When nothing seems to help, immunotherapy ("allergy shots") by an allergist, given over many months or years can be another consideration. Minimizing symptoms of allergies can go a long way in preventing secondary ear infections.

The good news is that as they get older, children become more resistant to upper respiratory tract and ear infections. The anatomy of the middle ear changes with time making it more difficult for bacteria to gain access. Children learn to wash their hands, blow their noses, and cover their coughs. Typically, the flood of ear infections tends to disappear by 1st grade making it much less likely for them to miss school due to illness.

Fever

"WHAT ABOUT A FEVER?"

High fevers in young children can be very scary. Every parent worries about possible convulsions (*febrile seizures*). Febrile seizures typically occur in children less than 5 years old. Two-thirds of young children with high fevers do not get convulsions. Those that do often have a family history of a close family member having had a childhood febrile seizure. Two-thirds of children that have had a febrile seizure do not go on to have another one. For those that do, there is prescription medication that can be given at the onset of fever for prevention.

If a child is less than 5 years old with a fever of 103 F or greater, (however the temperature is taken without adding or subtracting degrees), or if just "feels as though you could fry an egg on them", then proceed with the quickest way to lower the temperature - a *sponge bath*. *Do not use rubbing alcohol*. The fumes could make the child lethargic and appear much worse. Completely undress the child and place them in a tub of tepid water. Do not use cold water which promotes shivering which the body does to warm itself. Only use a small amount of water. One inch is all you need to keep wetting the child down.

The purpose is to promote evaporation of water from the skin which quickly causes heat loss. This can be facilitated by having a fan blowing or waving something like a magazine or newspaper to create a breeze against the wet skin. Within 15-20 minutes the temperature should drop below 103F. If not proceed to the ER.

High fevers are common in young children. The younger the child, the higher the febrile response. Most of the time, high fevers are caused by viral illnesses. Most viral illnesses tend to be less threatening than bacterial ones. The most common viral illness leading to a febrile seizure is *roseola.*

Typically, roseola occurs in children between 6 months to 5 yrs. of age. Fevers of 103-105F are common. Sudden onset of high fever in a relatively well appearing toddler is characteristic of *Roseola.* It is usually not associated with ear infections. The telltale indication of *roseola* is a rash that does not appear until after 1-4 days of intermittent high fevers. The fever suddenly goes away and only until then does the rash breaks out. The rash of roseola is "*maculopapular*" i.e. generalized small blotchy areas that are slightly bumpy and can be felt with your eyes closed. It is reddish pink and fades away over several days without treatment.

Reassuring is when the child looks well, smiling and is playful despite the high fever. When treated with fever reducers, the fever readily comes down. This is often referred to as a non-*toxic* appearance.

Be sure the child is drinking fluids ok and not dehydrated. Fever causes fluid loss which could lead to *dehydration* making the fever worse.

What is **Not Reassuring**:

- Any fever in an infant less than 2 months old no matter how slight needs to be evaluated ASAP.

- Any high fever associated with repeated vomiting. An upset child may vomit once just because they are upset, but more than once all bets are off. Too many very serious and life-threatening infections can present with no more than high fever and vomiting. Typically, the child looks ill.

- Any high fever that does not come down quickly, especially with an existing rash.

- Most concerning is a rash that looks pinpoint and cannot be felt with your eyes closed. These are tiny hemorrhages in the skin called *petechiae* and can

indicate a life-threatening infection, especially if the

petechia are below the upper chest.

Note: vomiting can cause tiny blood vessels to break in the

face, neck and upper chest, but not the lower body. Even more

frightening is the appearance of bleeding under the skin (*purpura*),

which could be a sign of life-threatening blood disorders or infection.

- *Any fever lasting greater than 5 days no matter how well a child appears should be medically evaluated.*

Vomiting

"My child won't stop vomiting"

This is a common call at night. Concerned parents typically do their best to prevent dehydration by pushing clear fluids or an electrolyte solution such as "Pedialyte". Unfortunately, the harder they try the worse the vomiting often gets.

The way to stop this is to not offer anything (not even a sip of water or a lick from a Popsicle) for 3 hrs. in order to give the irritated stomach a chance to rest. With protracted vomiting, the stomach becomes so irritable that the tiniest offering of fluid causes the stomach to cramp and continue to vomit.

Vomiting that continues despite having an empty stomach and being "NPO" (nothing by mouth) X 3 hrs., or any vomiting that recurs for more than 12 hrs., needs to be seen and evaluated. Typically, slow gradual reintroduction of clear fluids (or ideally an electrolyte solution such as "Pedialyte"), will remedy the situation.

An example would be to start with very small amounts like 1/2 oz. (= 15 ml=1 tbsp.). Wait 20 min. If tolerated increase to 1 oz., then 2 oz., 3 oz. and eventually 4 oz. while waiting 20 min. in between increases. If 4 oz. stays down, then it is safe to offer the child as much as they want. Until then, letting a child drink that much will typically lead to more vomiting.

Having significant *diarrhea* along with vomiting can actually be a good sign in that it can be an indication of a **viral gastroenteritis** (like rotavirus or *norovirus* [the "cruise ship virus"]) and not a surgical emergency. *Signs of blood* in the diarrhea or vomitus is concerning and needs prompt evaluation.

It's wise to continue clear fluids for the rest of the day and introduce soft bland foods the next day gradually progressing to a regular diet. Note that one drop of viral diarrhea contains *billions* of viruses and is *highly contagious*. More often than not it spreads to every household member. Hand sanitizers help but actual hand washing with soap and water works best to prevent its spread.

Vomiting by itself can be a sign of many very serious, life threatening conditions and surgical emergencies.

Worrisome:

- Any *"bilious"* vomiting, i.e. containing bile, in an *infant* (<6 months old) should be considered a surgical emergency until proven otherwise and evaluated urgently.

- *Vomiting with high fevers* also needs urgent evaluation.

- Vomiting that continues through the night into the following morning needs evaluation ASAP.

- Vomiting accompanied by *increasing abdominal pain* can be indicative of critical abdominal conditions (such as, but not limited to, appendicitis).

- Vomiting *with severe headache* should be considered indicative of serious neurologic conditions or infections until proven otherwise and needs prompt evaluation.

- *Cyclic vomiting* has many causes, some very serious. A thorough evaluation starting with a detailed history and physical exam followed by additional testing as indicated should be pursued.

- Intractable vomiting, not responsive to simple measures, often needs IV fluids and evaluation in an Emergency Room.

Vomiting should not be taken lightly. It often requires a detailed history and thorough exam to properly assess.

With infants, it is important to differentiate between actual vomiting vs an extreme episode of "spitting up". Spitting up is typically due to *gastroesophageal reflux (GER),* often related to position or motion on a full stomach.

Babies with *GER* look unaffected and happy. They are thriving and gaining weight well. Right after what appears to be a large amount of "vomiting" (typically all over their mother) they seem ready to take another feeding.

The babies that have just truly *vomited* look sick. They look as if their bellies hurt and are not anxious to eat right afterwards. Some of those babies have food allergies.

Babies that have "*projectile*" vomiting are very concerning. These are babies that look sick and often are losing weight. Most commonly they have an increasing obstruction just beyond the bottom of the

stomach known as *pyloric stenosis*. Their stomach works harder and

harder to push a feeding beyond its outlet but can't. Eventually their

stomach contents "explode" backwards as if being fired from a canon

traveling several feet through the air. Bowel movements may be fewer

or none at all. This condition usually appears between 4-8 wks. of age

and is treated surgically once dehydration and electrolyte imbalances

have been corrected.

Sudden Onset of Difficulty Breathing

This is also a frequent call in the middle of the night, especially in early fall and winter.

Worrisome: If the child is *leaning forward* to breath, *drooling* and *can't swallow* call **911** as this can be an indication of *epiglottis* an imminent life-threatening situation.

Difficulty breathing may present itself with rapid breathing (*tachypnea*), and *retractions* (where you can see prominent ribs, collar bones and accessory neck muscles), as a result of working hard to breathe. *Grunting* with each breath as you exhale is another sign often seen with serious forms of *pneumonia.* Any of these signs should prompt urgent evaluation.

More than likely, particularly in young children, a sudden onset of difficulty breathing is *croup*. This is a viral infection that affects the area below the *larynx* (the "voice box"). A hoarse, raspy, strained sounding noise ("*stridor*") is produced when the child takes in a breath.

The more anxious the child gets, the more difficult their breathing gets as they struggle to get in each breath.

This is opposite to *wheezing,* the noise made when exhaling. This is the sound made by children with *asthma* and *bronchiolitis.* Symptoms range from mild to severe with increasing labored breathing producing retractions, tachypnea, and difficult, prolonged exhaling. Croup typically comes on suddenly and at night. Both croup and bronchiolitis may be accompanied by fever.

What to do:

For suspected **croup**:

1. Don't panic. Your anxiety gets transferred to the child and makes matters worse. Hold the child to comfort him or her and hopefully relax their breathing. Next, steam up the bathroom using *HOT* water from the shower. Take the child (in your arms) into the bathroom (not the shower) and let them breathe the steam. This often gives dramatic relief.

2. If no better, take the child outside and let them breathe the chilly night air. This too can have dramatic results.

3. If still no better head to the Emergency Room with the windows open in the vehicle. Often by the time you arrive, things are much better, then you can turn around and head home.

4. If still no better proceed into the ER where specific medications can be administered either by inhalation via a nebulizer, by mouth or by injection. If unresponsive, other causes can be investigated. Croup is typically caused by a virus that runs a self-limited course lasting several days or as short as 24-48 hrs. Antibiotics are of no help in uncomplicated croup.

For **asthma:**

Flare ups often occur in the early fall when chilly nights lead to turning up the thermostat causing dust to circulate in the generated heat. This often looks like infection that is not responding to treatment.

1. Signs of labored breathing can sometimes be quickly relieved with albuterol, by nebulizer or inhaler (preferably using a "spacer" to improve delivery of the medication). An empty toilet paper roll can substitute for a spacer if one is not available.

2. If significant wheezing persists, call the doctor. Do not attempt to repeat the dose of albuterol without further instruction.

3. If breathing is still labored, proceed to Urgent Care or the Emergency Room without delay. Waiting too long allows symptoms to escalate to a point too extreme to easily reverse and may result in hospitalization.

Best methods of prevention: Heating systems, especially *forced hot air, stir* up accumulated dust from the warmer months. Often in mid-

October there can be a sudden onset of asthma in the middle of the night when the temperature drops and the furnace "kicks in".

Wet dusting, vacuuming in between the fins of baseboard heating elements, changing the furnace filter before the cold weather arrives and using a HEPA filter in the bedroom can make a difference. Eliminate any dust collectors in the bedroom. Avoid storing unessential items under the bed. Stuffed animals taken to bed can collect a lot of dust. Periodically toss them into the washing machine. Plastic covers on the mattress and pillow can also help to minimize dust exposure.

Using preventative medication just before an anticipated allergy season is a good measure. Major allergy seasons include dust- all year but especially in fall, tree pollen- (late winter early spring), grasses- (mid spring and summer) and ragweed "goldenrod"- (late summer).

When all else fails, seeing an allergist, getting allergy testing, medication and *immunotherapy* ("allergy shots") may help.

Not all wheezing is asthma. *Bronchiolitis* looks a lot like asthma. It is a viral infection usually caused by the *RSV virus*. It is highly contagious amongst young children and often progresses to moderate and severe respiratory distress especially in infants. This infection requires close office monitoring and can lead to hospitalization. Other serious conditions can look like bronchiolitis, asthma or croup and require further evaluation when not improving as expected.

Word of caution regarding inhalers

It is not uncommon to receive a call at night that "the asthma inhaler (sometimes referred to as a "puffer") ran out and we need a refill (i.e. *albuterol*). Children with *chronic asthma* should not rely on albuterol alone (via inhaler or nebulizer). It is a real temptation since albuterol typically gives immediate relief of wheezing, tightness in the chest and shortness of breath. The problem is that albuterol does not treat inflammation, just bronchial "spasm" (i.e. *bronchospasm*).

Prolonged symptoms, i.e. with *chronic / intermittent asthma*, are accompanied by increasing inflammation, swelling and narrowing of the airways, making albuterol less and less effective. Consequently, albuterol gets used more and more often with potential for

overuse.   Overuse of albuterol can lead to increased heart rate, blood

pressure and potentially cause life threatening *arrhythmias*.

The solution is treatment with anti-inflammatory medication

("*controllers*") such as inhaled steroids. Proper use is very safe and

avoids systemic absorption and serious side effects. Because its onset

of action is much slower than albuterol (but much longer duration), the

tendency is to go right to albuterol when getting into trouble. You

should never use albuterol more frequently than directed. If you feel the

need to use albuterol more often than prescribed you should be calling

the doctor.

Diarrhea

Diarrhea is an extremely common problem most often due to common viruses. Typically (but not always) there is no fever, and no blood in the stool. Sometimes there is vomiting but not lasting > 12 hrs. Watery explosive stools can last up to 7-10 days. The younger the child the longer it can last. An affected adult may have symptoms for 12-24 hrs. In a school age child, it may last for a few days, but in an infant, it can last for almost 2 wks. With improvement the number of stools start to decline before the watery, explosive consistency improves. A return to "normal" for an infant may mean 2-3 stools per day of loose to mushy consistency. Sometimes this becomes a "new normal" for several weeks and even a few months. High fevers and even a slight streak or hint of blood in the stool can indicate a more serious infection such as salmonella and should prompt further evaluation. Prolonged diarrhea greater than 3 weeks also needs evaluation.

Treatment is focused around preventing dehydration and allowing it to run its course without making matters worse. Diarrhea is usually accompanied by transient *lactose intolerance.* Therefore, it is wise to avoid regular milk and dairy products containing lactose until a normal stool pattern has been reestablished.

Treatment for severe watery diarrhea is best by giving nothing but clear fluids (ideally an electrolyte solution such as "Pedialyte") for 24 hrs. The following day one can introduce a "BRAT" diet to children on whole foods. This would include Bananas, Rice or Rice cereal, Apple sauce, and Toast. For older children think the 3 B's: Boiled, Broiled and Baked. Avoid greasy fried foods, spicy foods or foods considered to be high in "roughage".

Infants less than 6 months of age merit special consideration. If breastfeeding, continue to nurse but also give supplemental Pedialyte between feedings. For formula fed babies it is good to temporarily switch to a lactose free or soy formula until things settle down. For extreme, persistent, watery diarrhea, feeding with an "elemental" formula such as *Nutramigen* or *Alimentum* may turn things around.

Close medical follow-up is essential. Dehydration and more serious causes need to be ruled-out.

Chronic diarrhea necessitates a medical evaluation. Before pursuing further evaluation make sure lactose has been eliminated from the diet as well as juices and sugary drinks. The high concentrations of sugars (sucrose and fructose) can cause the bowel to attempt to dilute them, secreting more fluid into the bowel causing more diarrhea. This is known as *osmotic diarrhea* and can be prevented by replacing these products with plain water or lactose free milk.

.

Crying

"WHAT SHOULD I DO WHEN MY BABY IS CRYING DURING THE

NIGHT?"

First, rule out the obvious. Is it time for a feeding? Is the diaper wet? If crying persists, check on the baby without turning the lights on. Make sure there is nothing striking like having an extremity stuck between the bars of a crib. If the crying still persists, pick the baby up in the dark. DO NOT TURN ON THE LIGHTS. If the crying stops, bad things are typically ruled out. All babies love to be held. They cannot be held 24/7. You are not being a terrible parent if you say, "night-time is for sleeping so it's time to go back to bed". DO NOT take the baby to bed with you. First there is the risk of falling asleep and rolling over onto the baby causing injury or suffocation. Second you create a bad habit that becomes increasingly more difficult to break with time and stresses marital life.

If the crying still persists, turn on the lights, totally undress the baby and get a good look at everything from top to bottom. The cause may then become apparent such as the unusual finding of a *tourniquet syndrome* where a long hair falls into "footie" pajamas or the diaper and becomes wrapped around an appendage such as a toe, finger or even a penis.

Night-time crying can be due to "gas pains" from swallowed air, difficulty burping, or difficulty digesting feedings such as certain formulas containing lactose.

Use caution when feeding an infant with its stomach in an *inverted position.* This can occur when nursing with the baby lying alongside of its mother whose elbow is leaning into the bed. The baby's head can inadvertently become lower than its stomach. In this position swallowed air quickly floats to the "top" which is the "bottom" of the baby's inverted stomach and readily passes into the bowel before there is a chance to be burped up.

Jiggling or bouncing on your knee can bring up the air "bubble". Vibrations from a ride in the car or even placing in a carrier seat on top of the washing machine while running a load of laundry can help.

Sometimes a hot water bottle (with *warm* water) placed on the belly or placing the baby in a tub of warm water can help. The later may first produce a momentary increase in crying as the internal gas expands but shortly thereafter "bubbles" float up through the tub water and the gas pains are relieved.

"Gas drops" (i.e. *simethicone)* are helpful. These are not absorbed and work on the surface tension of the gas bubbles breaking them up into tiny ones that are easier to pass.

Make sure there is no constipation. An infant *glycerin suppository* may trigger a bowel movement and make for a happier baby. If all else fails and the crying becomes relentless and inconsolable it is time to head to the Emergency Room. Babies that are fussy all the time, both day and night, may have *gastroesophageal reflux* as well as several other conditions that are best evaluated during the day at the doctor's

office.

The Common Cold

"HOW CAN YOU TELL WHEN A COLD NEEDS TO BE TREATED?"

Most *colds (URI's) last 7-10 days.* They are due to cold viruses which do not respond to antibiotics. Typically, they present with a runny nose of clear mucus but sometimes can start out with cloudy mucus. After 5-7 days there should be some signs of improvement.

Be concerned if:

- you are not seeing improvement when expected.
- seeing a fever when there had been none to begin with.
- the mucous is changing to a thick cloudy mucus when it was initially clear.
- after a week when you would expect to see some sign of improvement or at least no sign of getting worse, it's not.
- developing increasing cough, looking sicker or just lasting longer than 2 weeks. At this point it is time to get things

checked out. Antibiotics are likely indicated for a secondary bacterial infection.

Often times a secondary bacterial sinus infection develops. Infants and young children do not get sinus infections like adults because their sinuses are still developing. Prior to school age children typically have only one set of sinuses- the *ethmoid sinuses*. These sit directly behind the bridge of the nose adjacent to the tear ducts. When they become infected (ethmoid sinusitis) it is common to see a "goopy" discharge from a tear duct. It may look like *conjunctivitis (pink eye)* but upon close inspection the white of the eye is not pink or red. Instead the tear sac may have become infected (*dacryocystitis*). Infection in the ethmoid sinuses can easily spread to the middle ear as well as the tear ducts.

It is common for parents to request eye drops to treat "conjunctivitis". I would *caution* against not having the child seen in the office. What happens when antibiotic eye drops are applied, the eye discharge may then appear clear, but an accompanying ear infection goes undetected. Complications could easily develop.

Infection of the ethmoid sinuses can easily spread to the surrounding tissue around the eye and orbit producing *periorbital cellulitis*. This is a very serious complication often requiring hospitalization.

Common bacteria that cause sinus and ear infections such as haemophilus influenza and pneumococcus, on rare occasion, can spread into the bloodstream, bones, joints, brain and surrounding tissue, potentially becoming life threatening.   Fortunately, these complications are very unusual beyond 6 years of age. Early childhood immunizations greatly help in preventing them.

Part II: Frequent Summer Concerns and Precautions

Ticks

"AT BATH TIME TONIGHT WE FOUND AN ATTACHED TICK,

WHAT SHOULD WE DO?"

First remove the tick. Avoid squeezing the body of the tick with tweezers. This could inoculate organisms into the skin that cause diseases such as Lyme Disease commonly found in New England. The best way to remove a tick is to grab it in front of its head and give it a tug. The pincers typically do not release but instead take with it a tiny piece of skin leaving a tiny speck of a wound in the skin. Clean this with soap and water then apply a triple antibiotic ointment such as "Neosporin". The concerning tick is the deer tick, which is tiny, about the size of the head of a common pin. To produce Lyme Disease the tick needs to remain attached for at least 48-72 hrs. The area needs to be observed for the next 7-14 days. Concerning would be the development of a pimple like inflammation at the bite site which later develops into a spreading red rash becoming pale in the center. This is the "bull's eye" rash of *erythema migrans* characteristic of Lyme Disease. Later findings can produce a swollen large joint like the knee as well as a multitude of other symptoms. Fortunately, most ticks are discovered before they have a chance to produce infection.

More common are problems resulting from the attempted tick removal at home. It is common for pincer parts to remain in the skin. Repeated attempts at trying to remove "all of the tick" often lead to secondary trauma and localized infection caused by surface bacteria such as a staph.

The best and easiest way to remove ticks is with a device called "TICKED OFF" or similar devices. These are very inexpensive and found in most pharmacies and pet stores. Remember to protect kids using an insect repellent containing DEET (<40% strength) and check daily even if your kids have only been playing on the front lawn.

Skin Issues

Sunburn:

Don't forget the sunscreen and reapply it periodically. Remember the best sun protection for babies is SHADE. A baby's skin is extremely sensitive. UV rays can penetrate through the clouds on overcast, cloudy days and still produce sunburn even to the extent of a blistered second - degree burn.

Contact Dermatitis:

Know how to identify *poison ivy* (figure 2) which can be found almost anywhere and is very prevalent in the North East. "IVY BLOCK" is a product that can be used to protect against accidental contact with the plant. Wash thoroughly ASAP following any accidental contact. It can take up to 7 days for the extremely itchy rash to break out after contact. 1% topical hydrocortisone and calamine lotion as well as several other OTC (over the counter) products can be helpful. When oozing and blisters develop OTC *burro solution* can be soothing and help dry them up. Moderate to severe involvement should be treated in your doctor's office. Secondary infection can also develop requiring additional treatment.

Poison Ivy

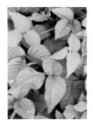

Figure 2

Insect bites:
    Watch out for biting insects. No-see-ums, black flies and mosquitoes typically become active when the sun goes down. Don't forget the insect repellent. DEET is the ingredient that works far better than citronella and other natural products. Avoid products containing >40% DEET.

Treat *itching* with over the counter (OTC) 1% hydrocortisone ointment or cream. Calamine lotion can be helpful as well as oral *Benadryl.* Itching and scratching commonly lead to impetigo and other skin infections. These can lead to other complications including severe kidney disease (*acute streptococcal glomerulonephritis*) and *cellulitis.*

Neosporin or other OTC triple antibiotic ointments should be applied at the first signs of inflammation. Clean all scratches and apply the topical antibiotic. Clean open dirty cuts with *hydrogen peroxide.* Keep plenty of BAND-AIDS on hand. Light summer clothing with long sleeves and long pants can help minimize scratching.

Bee stings:
Often cause localized redness and swelling. Most do not go on to life threatening anaphylaxis. If there is a known bee sting allergy, you should immediately administer injectable epinephrine (e.g. EPIPEN) *first* and then BENADRYL. DON'T wait to see if symptoms are going to develop. Remember, the duration of this injection is short lasting and

should be repeated every 15-20 min while awaiting a response to a 911 call.

To avoid bee stings, avoid areas that attract bees such as trash cans around picnic areas and flowers. Avoid flowery print clothing. You do not want to look or smell like a flower. Some bees make their nests in the ground and in pine needles. Keep ankles covered in these areas. Consulting an allergist to test for the specific type of bee allergy and the possibility of desensitization with immunotherapy ("allergy shots") is worth considering.

A *severe localized skin reaction* to a bee sting can be quite extensive and not be a true anaphylactic reaction. The distinction is that it is contiguous with the site of the bite. It does not cause hives or swelling in areas not connected to the bite such as with multiple hives. It is not an allergy and not a life-threatening reaction.

An *anaphylactic reaction* is life threatening and may produce generalized hives, areas of redness and swelling not contiguous with the site of the sting, swelling of the tongue, difficulty breathing, swallowing and symptoms affecting areas other than the skin.

REMEMBER IMMEDIATE Epi-Pen THEN 911! (Repeat Epi-pen in 15 min if an ambulance has not arrived yet).

Part III: Common Concerning Incidents

Animal Related Issues

Animal Bites:
Animal bites can be a much more complicated situation. First wash the area then apply a topical antibiotic. Next consider the potential for *rabies exposure.* Newborn wild animals may seem cute but can be carrying rabies without initially looking or acting ill. They should never be picked up without a minimum of 10 days observation for signs of rabies. Of particular high risk, are baby raccoons and feral kittens, not to

mention stray cats. The biting animal should always be quarantined for 10 days and watched for signs of rabies if not euthanized and examined immediately for rabies. If this is not possible you should assume the worse and get rabies prophylaxis.

Rabies is essentially 100% fatal. There is a very safe and effective vaccine to prevent the development of rabies ASAP following possible exposure. This prophylactic vaccine is extremely expensive, not typically found in a private office, but is available in an emergency room. It involves 1 injection of Rabies Immune Globulin + 4 injections of Rabies Vaccine over 14 days.

Bat strain rabies have been found in patients who have died from rabies with no signs of a bite. For that reason, extra caution should be observed if waking up with a bat flying around in a child's bedroom. It should be assumed that the bat could have landed on the face or an exposed extremity. Rabies prophylaxis is indicated in this situation unless the bat is tested and found not to have rabies.

Stray and domestic animals which have bitten a child should be reported to the local animal control officer unless it is your own or you can be assured that if it becomes ill within 10 days you will be notified immediately.

Cat Scratches:

Kittens (not mature cats) are capable of transmitting *Cat Scratch Disease* with their needle like claws. Wash the scratches immediately and apply a topical antibiotic. If the area becomes inflamed or a swollen lymph node develops seek medical attention. Typically, over several days to weeks an alarmingly large lymph node will develop almost the size of a golf ball. The armpit, neck or groin are the areas where it is most often likely to develop depending on its proximity to the scratch.

Human Bites:

Typically, these are from a teething toddler. These are capable of producing serious infection particularly if they break the skin. They need the same immediate attention as animal bites, i.e. soap and water, topical antibiotic and medical attention if there is an open wound or signs of infection are developing i.e. redness, increasing warmth or tenderness.

Tetanus: All open wounds and puncture wounds have the potential for developing *tetanus* which is a ubiquitous organism found in the soil. Wounds should be cleaned with mild soap and water ASAP. Hydrogen peroxide is particularly helpful in cleaning puncture wounds. It is essential to keep tetanus immunizations up to date. If not, one should be administered within 24 hrs. of the injury.

Head Injuries

Head injuries are extremely common and represent a fair number of afterhours calls. Extreme injuries are immediate 911 calls. All others cause great concern especially when the evening approaches.

Head injuries in babies often occur when a baby is placed on a bed momentarily and suddenly rolls off onto a hard surface floor. Babies should not be taken to bed with you because of serious risk of injuries and suffocation.

Concerning is when a baby develops a swelling on the head, a bulging soft spot (*fontanelle*), acts lethargic, has inconsolable crying, becomes extremely irritable, is not moving an extremity or is vomiting. These are signs of great concern and need emergency evaluation. Sometimes a baby will fall down several stairs in its mother's arms as she trips. Often the baby is protected by the mother's body, immediately cries and appears normal shortly after with none of the concerning signs present. This would be **reassuring**.

A word of caution: This type of fall poses an increased risk of an extremity fracture. If close inspection is not reassuring, emergency evaluation is indicated.

If all seems well, observe. Avoid an immediate feeding which may be vomited and prompt an ER visit that could have been avoided. After prolonged crying an infant or child might normally want to sleep. This is ok if everything seems well. Just be sure to wake the infant or child every couple of hours to make sure they respond appropriately and seem well oriented.

Looking for changes in the *size of the pupils* can be helpful but this is often a late sign of a serious head injury and preceded by many of the concerning signs already mentioned. What you would be looking for would be *a very obvious difference*, not something subtle requiring repeated inspections.

Toddlers and preschoolers sometimes collide heads or run into a door or post. The result is often a golf ball size swelling on the forehead the "pops up" immediately. Loose tissue in this area allows for soft tissue fluid to collect quickly. The swelling should come down just as quickly with an application of an ice pack or "frozen peas". Peas or other small vegetables like corn can readily conform to the shape of the swelling. If it does not come down and persists into the next day, or at any time concerning symptoms develop seek further evaluation.

School age children and teens tend to have more serious injuries, usually sports related. Common are helmet to helmet collisions in football. Most common sports related head injuries occur with hockey, soccer, stick injuries in field hockey and lacrosse, falling backwards onto ice, pole vaulting, horseback riding to name a few. The mechanism of injury, force and height involved can indicate the severity of injury.

On site evaluation should include mental status and orientation. Ask questions like what's your name, where are you, what day is it, etc. Being disoriented, "having your bell rung" or even momentary loss of consciousness are signs of a *concussion* at the least. The player should sit out the remainder of the game and be closely observed. Loss of memory for recent events (*retrograde amnesia*), loss of consciousness beyond momentary, vomiting, severe headache, numbness, weakness, persistent dizziness and lethargy are very concerning and should have prompt if not urgent medical evaluation. All concussions should be medically evaluated and monitored until resolved with restrictions in activities as indicated.

Accidental Ingestions

Parents should always have this number readily available:

***National Poison Control Hotline** 24 hrs./day*

1-800-222-1222

Children are very curious and tend to put anything and everything in their mouth. All the "child proofing" in the world can never replace the need to always keep a close eye on them. Children explore with their mouths. There are typically no shortages of hazardous chemicals and toxic medications in the home. Safety cabinet locks can be undone. Some safety caps on medications can be bitten off. Children get creative exploring "out of reach items". They easily climb up cabinet draws like rungs on a ladder to reach high shelves or to get on to a countertop with access from there. They look for objects to climb up on to reach what you thought were out of reach items. You cannot be too cautious. Not all poisons are good to induce vomiting and may lead to life threatening complications. Calling Poison Control is the quickest and best action to take.

Choking:

In children (not infants) the *Heimlich maneuver* can be lifesaving and every parent should be familiar with it. In infants this maneuver has the potential of causing internal abdominal injury. Do not sit a child upright and administer a blow between their shoulder blades as this may cause a small object to drop down and lodge deeper in the throat or lungs. Placing them across your lap with their head lower than their body or actually holding them upside down then applying a blow between the shoulder blades is ok and can be effective. A "finger sweep" to the back of the throat should be a last desperate effort. It is easy to scratch or lacerate the soft palate and tissues in the back of the throat with a fingernail. This can lead to critical complications such as a *retropharyngeal abscess*. Use this procedure when all else fails.

With any critical situation a 911 call should always be made before considering a call to the doctor. Never hesitate to call the pediatrician when concerned with a serious issue at night. Hopefully lesser problems and concerns are addressed during the daytime. Night call constitutes a significant part of a pediatrician's life. Medical problems always seem to get worse at night along with heightened parental concerns when dealing with an ill infant or child.

I hope The Little Jeffrey Book with its collection of discussions that I had shared with many parents in the middle of the night (with some diversion on related issues) helps to get parents through those nights that keep them (and often their pediatrician) up at night.

About the author

Dr. David A. Avila, D.O., FACOP, FAAP, is Founder and past president of Pediatric Professional Associates in Methuen, Massachusetts, past chief of the departments of pediatrics at Lawrence General Hospital in Lawrence, MA and Holy Family Hospital in Methuen, MA. Practiced Neonatal and Pediatric intensive care as well as general pediatrics at Grandview Hospital and Children's Hospital both of Dayton, Ohio before returning to Massachusetts where he practiced most of his 40 years in primary care Pediatrics. He was very active in numerous hospital committees, the local Methuen Board of Health, mentored numerous premed and medical students. Awarded the Massachusetts Pride in Medicine Award in 1989 and in 2012 was the recipient of the St. Luke's Award from Holy Family Hospital in

Methuen, MA. He lived with his wife and three daughters in southern

NH and retired in Sept. of 2017. He now spends winters in Arizona and

summers in NH and VT.

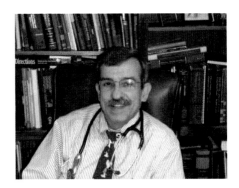

Figure 3 "Dr. Dave"

POSTSCRIPT

Unfortunately for some parents, what keeps them up in the middle of the night are problems which seem insurmountable, leaving them feeling helpless with a sense of hopelessness. There are those children with suicidal behaviors, anger, aggressiveness, self-destructive behaviors, and other behaviors that impede with functioning at home and school.

When everyone else has given up on the most troubled of kids, there is BOYS TOWN. At BOYS TOWN they believe in not giving up on any child, that every child deserves a second chance, and an opportunity to reach their full potential. They work closely with parents and children, including girls since 1979. Their mission is saving children and healing families. They also work with children who are suffering from bullying, abuse, abandonment, violence and addiction.

There are numerous locations beyond the main BOYS TOWN campus in Nebraska, each offering its own set of Child and family services.

For parents and kids needing help in a crisis situation, help is available 24 hr./day by calling the

BOYS TOWN CRISIS HOTLINE:

1-800–448-3000

They never give up on kids.

*A portion of the proceeds from every *The Little Jeffrey Book* will be donated to BOYS TOWN.

"We spend so little time in our lives as children, yet it is the most important time in our lives". – Dr. Avila

Learn more at boystown.org

Kids deserve to be kids!

Acknowledgements:

Editing: MacKenzie Michaud, Judy De Luca

Technical support: Jennifer Copp

Index

Made in the USA
San Bernardino, CA
01 March 2020

65187852R00042